"Leah has created a book of valuable information based on her many years at the bedside, supporting patients at the end of life and comforting their caregivers. The content of this book reflects the questions that most every caregiver asks and the answers she has provided are both practical, and also sacred, respecting the end of life as indeed a sacred time."

—Betty Ferrell PhD, FAAN, FPCN, CHPN
Professor, City of Hope Medical Center
Director, the End of Life Nursing Education Consortium (ELNEC) project

"I first read Leah's book nine years ago when my mother was passing away. It answered so many of my questions and helped me understand the process of her passing. Last September when my husband was dying, I re-read her book, and shared it with many family members. Again, her book was an invaluable help to me, and my family. We all feel that anyone losing a loved on should have this information. Hospice was helpful, but Leah's book led us to a deeper understanding of the of the process of his passing."

—Nancy Dorey

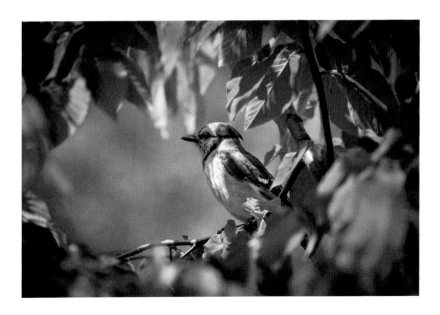

The Journey Back - Changes at the End of Life

Leah Middleton RN, CHPN

Balboa Press books may be ordered through booksellers or by contacting:

Balboa Press
A Division of Hay House
1663 Liberty Drive
Bloomington, IN 47403
www.balboapress.com
844-682-1282

Because of the dynamic nature of the Internet, any web addresses or links contained in this book may have changed since publication and may no longer be valid. The views expressed in this work are solely those of the author and do not necessarily reflect the views of the publisher, and the publisher hereby disclaims any responsibility for them.

Any people depicted in stock imagery provided by Getty Images are models, and such images are being used for illustrative purposes only.
Certain stock imagery © Getty Images.

ISBN: 979-8-7652-5309-0 (sc)
ISBN: 979-8-7652-5310-6 (e)

Print information available on the last page.

Balboa Press rev. date: 06/27/2024

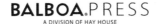

CONTENTS

INTRODUCTION

What is life? It is truly a mystery. We really do not know what lies ahead, we only know each moment as we experience it. This includes our end of life and this process is a mystery as well.

We are labored into life and we have to labor out of life. Labor is a process of somewhat predictable events. We often have heard the phrase "There is a light at the end of every tunnel." There are many, many references to this throughout life. I believe it couldn't be truer than with birth and death. Each journey holds the mystery to the cycle of life.

When we are told that the end of our life, or the life of someone we love, is near, our grief process begins. There are more questions, more fears, and more unknowns. This is a time when support from those who work with end-of-life issues can be helpful and reassuring. It is time to consider Hospice support.

Hospice staff, perhaps a nurse, social worker, or chaplain, can talk with you and explain, in common language, the changes you or your loved one may experience at the end of life. This may be a difficult conversation for you to have. You will find that those helping you through Hospice services will be compassionate and understanding with your needs and feelings.

The information listed on the following pages will, hopefully, be helpful to all who are involved in this journey. The information in this book is to help you become more aware of the changes that may occur at the end of life. All of them are changes that have been designed by nature to guide us out of life. My hope is that by knowing what you might expect, you will not be as alarmed when they occur and will feel more comfortable with the process at hand.

People vary greatly; as in life, so as in death. Some people have all and some only a few of the changes discussed on the following pages. With a natural dying process, most of these "predictable events" will occur. However, there is the "unpredictable". Those are the unique qualities we each hold as individuals.

SLEEPING

As the end of life approaches, you will notice your loved one sleeps more and more. This is normal. When they are awake, try to make this quality time. They may be quiet or talkative, restless or subdued. You may not be able to make any sense out of what they are saying as they often are coming out of a dream state.

It may also be that they do not sleep at night. This can be very tiring and upsetting. It is important for the caregiver to take care of themselves and you <u>must</u> have sleep; at least four hours straight sleep is advised. So, get help and take shifts if necessary. Another thing that can make a difference is an intercom, especially if you are not sleeping in the same room. Not having to sleep with "your ears open" can allow you to sleep more deeply.

FOOD

Your loved one may refuse food, some or even most of the time. They may only take a bite or two of the "special" dish or their "favorite" food that they told you they wanted. Loss of appetite is to be expected. Swallowing may be a problem. Pain medications slow down the digestive system which can lead to decreased appetite and slower bowel activity, i.e. constipation.

Weight loss can tighten the muscles in the neck making it harder to swallow. Offer food and if they are hungry, they will eat. If they are choking when they swallow, this may cause food to enter the airway and go into the lungs, possibly causing an aspiration pneumonia. Food should NOT be forced as vomiting may occur. Pureed food or protein shakes may be swallowed easier and lessen the possibility of choking. Baby food can also be an alternative.

If they don't want to eat, honor their wishes; you will not be starving them. A body that is shutting down does not need food. It is very hard to stand by and let it be when you want to be doing everything you can to keep them comfortable. Forcing food on them can actually cause them discomfort. We are nurturing by nature, so this can be a very hard thing to do. Trust that you are responding to their needs.

FLUIDS

Fluids may also be refused. As long as they are rouseable, offer liquids to them. When sucking through a straw becomes too difficult, use the straw like a pipette and place a small amount of liquid on their tongue or the side of their mouth. Keeping the mouth moist help to prevent the saliva from drying and sticking to the inside of the mouth. A toothette or swab or even a damp cloth can be used to moisten and/or clean their mouth. I consider oral hygiene as a comfort measure.

Have the head of the bed up to help prevent choking. Observe their ability to swallow. Again, if they are not swallowing well and are choking, just as with food, caution is necessary. Sometimes adding a little lemon to the water or giving water that is warm or at room temperature rather than cold can be swallowed easier.

Dehydration is a normal part of the dying process. It is generally painless. It may, however, cause confusion. To rehydrate a dying body only makes them have to dehydrate again. Rehydration, such as the use of intravenous fluids, can become an added burden to the heart. This may cause edema (swelling) in the hands and feet.

Continued lack of fluids will also cause decreased urination and the color may become a dark yellow. As the other organs slow down their function, the urine gets darker. This process generally does not cause pain. However, if this pain is new, especially when they urinate, it may be a urinary tract infection. This should be reported to your nurse or doctor. Antibiotics can be a comfort measure.

SWALLOWING

As mentioned before, difficulty swallowing often occurs towards the end of life as the muscles tighten in the neck and secretions thicken with dehydration. Moistening the mouth and throat with a small amount of liquid before giving food or medications can help facilitate swallowing. When pills can no longer be swallowed whole, crushing them and putting them in pudding or applesauce or other easy-to-swallow food may aid the swallowing process.

It is <u>very important</u> **NOT** to crush time-released medications. If you have any questions about medications, please call your nurse or doctor. Liquid or topical pain medications can be substituted for tablets or capsules. It is important to not stop any medication, especially pain medication, without first talking with the nurse or doctor.

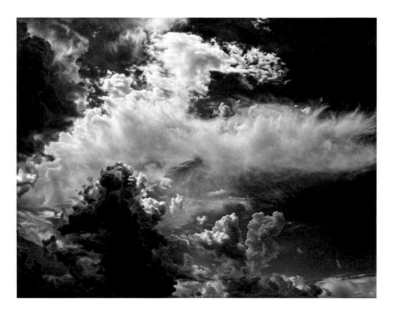

URINATION

Attends, Depends, "adult" diapers, briefs; they go by many names, but they are all used for the incontinence that can occur at the end of life or when they can no longer stand to get to the bedside commode. Occasionally, external or internal catheters may be necessary. Your Hospice nurse will be evaluating your loved one and will know what will be the most appropriate way to manage their incontinence. Chux and washable pads are also very convenient for caregivers. Often Hospice can often provide you with these items.

As mentioned before, the urine may change to a darker color and the amount and frequency may decrease. Keeping the skin clean and dry of urine is very important in preventing skin irritation and breakdown.

For a person with a history of urinary tract infections, it is not uncommon to have them reoccur. If there is no discomfort or fever, often antibiotics are not given. Again, antibiotics can be a comfort measure. You and your care provider will decide what would be best.

BOWEL FUNCTION

This can be a major problem as constipation is a usual side effect of pain medications. Lack of physical activity and decreased fluid and food intake can also add to the slowing of the bowel. A bowel regime is always advised. It could be as simple as warm prune juice in the morning or a stool softener at bedtime. Bowel care can also get quite complex using laxatives and softeners several times a day. Occasionally, diarrhea can be a bowel problem. Over-the-counter Immodium is worth having on hand. The Hospice nurse will be routinely monitoring bowel function and adjusting the regime accordingly. Whenever you are concerned, there is someone on-call to assist you.

"THE DEATH RATTLE"

You hear it talked about, but what is it? It occurs when fluids and mucous gather deep at the back of the throat and get thick and sticky causing them to cling to the back of the throat. When they can no longer be cleared by coughing or swallowing, it causes a rattling sound. Mouth breathing, which is very common at the end of life, can exacerbate the death rattle. Sometimes the rattle is faint and other times they can get quite loud. These secretions cannot be suctioned out as they are too far back in the throat. The "death rattle" sometimes, but not always, happens just before someone dies. There is a drug intervention that may help to dry excessive secretions. Contact your nurse or doctor.

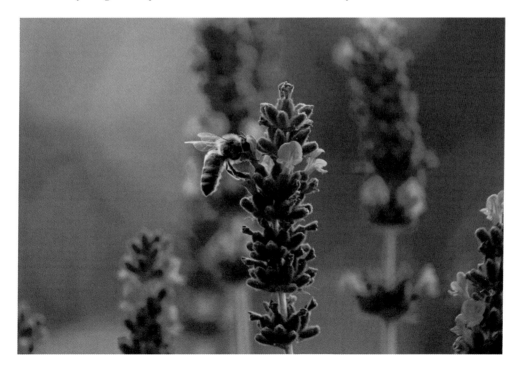

BODY CHANGES

-EXTREMITIES – Often towards the end of life you will notice that your loved ones hands and/or feet may become cool or even quite cold. There may be a bluish-red patchy look to the skin that may extend up the arms or legs. This is called mottling and happens as the circulation is slowing down. If they are complaining of being cold, try loose socks or extra blankets. Blankets can be warmed by running them in the dryer for a short time. It is advised not to use electric blankets, heating pads or hot water bottles as they may burn or injure fragile skin.

You may also notice swelling in the hands, arms, feet and/or legs. This is caused by the many changes that are occurring as the body labors out of life. Sometimes elevating the extremity on a pillow may help.

-BODY/SKIN- The body surface may become covered with a cool, damp, perspiration. Light weight blankets or sheets may help absorb this wetness and aid in keeping your loved one dry. Using powders or cornstarch is **not** recommended as they can cake and possibly trap fungus, like yeast. Using a hair dryer on low or warm can also aid in drying the skin. If you notice redness, especially in creases, you may apply an anti-fungal cream or protective barrier cream around the area. Be sure to inform your nurse of any changes to the skin. Having a home health aide to assist with personal care serves to maintain adequate hygiene, plus it gives a weary caregiver a break. It is a service that Hospice can provide to you.

With disease involving the liver, a condition called "jaundice" may occur. Jaundice is a yellow coloring of the skin and/or whites of the eyes. Occasionally, the skin may become orange or even brown. This can also be accompanied by mental confusion. Contact your Hospice nurse or doctor should these changes occur.

The body of a dying person is usually lying on their back. The head is tipped back slightly and the jaw is dropped. The eyes are often slightly open and may be looking upward. It is as though the openings of the face where our senses are located, are the portals through which the spirit leaves. I have found it interesting that when my Catholic patients receive last rites, the senses are anointed with oil.

Occasionally there is a fruity odor to the breath and/or skin. As the organs start shutting down and the metabolism changes, toxins are not being cleared in the usual way. The way the effects of these changes are noticed is by odor that comes through the pores of the skin and the breath.

-TURNING- With decreased nutrition, weight loss and/or dehydration, the skin and muscles become very thin. When a body is left in one position without movement for more than a couple hours, there is increased risk for developing pressure sores. The bones are heavy and push against these thinning tissues, cutting off circulation. Without the nutrition of the blood, the area dies and creates a sore. This process can happen in just a couple of hours. If you should notice redness over bony areas, Bag Balm may help. The best medicine, however, is turning. Once a sore has developed, they can be very hard to heal. They are also painful.

To help prevent pressure sores from developing, regular turning is advised. Every three to four hours is recommended. Generally turning from the back to one side and then the other side is the routine. Using a foam pad may delay skin breakdown, but, again, turning is the best medicine, even with the pad. Others pads such as alternating pressure mattresses and gel mattresses may be necessary. Your nurse will determine what would be the best choice.

The nurse or home health aide will teach you turning and positioning techniques. They will also be asking about your loved one's skin. Are there red areas or open sores? It is important to notify the nurse when you notice a change in your loved one's skin. The places to look are the tail bone, spine, hips, heels and, occasionally, the shoulders. Propping the ankles up on a pillow or using heel protectors can help prevent pressure to the heels. A foot guard can be used to keep the weight of the covers from pressing down on the feet.

MENTAL CONFUSION

As time goes on, your loved one may become confused as to time, surroundings and recognition of family and friends. This can be confusing and distressing to those around the person, but it is usually a normal occurrence at the end-stages of life. Reassuring your loved one that they are with people who love them and that they are being safely cared for, should be calming and reassuring. (See Restlessness)

Try not to downplay or negate what your loved one is saying, even though it may make no sense to you. They often wake up in a dream state and are confused to their reality. You can try to help them reorient themselves; but, if you can't, you can't. It is just part of their process, their journey, and you have done your best.

Occasionally, they may talk or call out to someone. It may be a deceased relative or a friend or a pet, or even new friends. When someone is in their transition state, their perception is different than ours. I liken it to microwaves; you can't see them, but you know they are there when the microwave cooks you food. When they are in this state, reassure them that "whomever" is there waiting to take their hand when they are ready, or whatever seems relevant at the moment. Your calm and caring presence should be soothing to them.

RESTLESSNESS

Sometimes referred to as "terminal agitation," restlessness can signal many things; low oxygen levels, discomfort, anxiety, or even pain. Comfort measures, such as keeping the oxygen on if you have it, or getting it if it is needed, and/or medications for agitation or pain, may be necessary to help decrease symptoms.

However, it may not be any of the above but simply that they are trying to leave their body, get out of their skin. They try to take off everything: clothing, oxygen, sometimes pull at indwelling catheters or their briefs, and/or are incontinent of urine and/or stool. They may want to "travel": get up and walk when they can't, they may insist they need to go to the bus or train or boat, or even drive the car. They may want to put on their clothes because they want to "go home." There can also be a constant need to go to the bathroom. These activities can cause caregivers distress and can be very tiring. Having someone to relieve you can be essential to your well-being. If a friend has offered to help you, take them up on it. There is also the Hospice volunteer that can come in so you can go take a well-deserved rest.

What may appear distressing to you as the caregiver may not be as distressing to your loved one. Labor is hard work. This activity can take hours or days. It is our human nature to take on another's suffering, or what appears to be suffering. Your loved one is not as affected by these occurrences as you might be. Having a medication for anxiety can help everyone. You can try holding their hand, having soft music playing, using the oxygen, and staying calm. These are just some of the ways to help you get through this often difficult part of their journey, the "birthing" out of life. Hospice is there to help you with these stressful times.

Occasionally along this journey your loved one may encounter demons or bugs or mean people. I have found that if you have them tell those "obstacles" to get out of their way because they have a better place to go, it often does get them to go away. You may want to discuss this with your nurse or doctor.

They may want you to try medication to help. If these symptoms persist, remember, "this too, shall pass." This is also a time where more than one caregiver may be necessary.

Another interesting occurrence that may happen is what I call "reaching and picking." Your loved one may hold their arms out, sometimes for long periods of time. Sometimes they "pick at the air." They may even want you to help them by holding their arm, or their back, if they are trying to sit up. They may also be scanning the ceiling, generally from left to right. They may even talk to "whomever." All you can do is go along with it. Again, it is part of their journey.

My grandmother told me, when she was dying and going through this experience, that "they" were giving her "the pieces" to her golden cord. Once she had some of "the pieces," she would move her fingers as though she was braiding. My job was to hold her arm up so she could reach them. She did this for 18 hours! I have had many other Hospice patients with similar experiences. It is quite amazing, even magical.

LEVEL OF CONSCIOUSNESS

When your loved one sleeps all of the time but you can rouse them by turning them or saying their name, this state is referred to as semi-comatose. They may even take their pill and go back to sleep. When they are not rouseable, this is comatose. This state may last several days or only several minutes. It may not happen at all and they will talk with you until their very last breath. More often, there is a time when they stop verbalizing but may still acknowledge you with their eyes or a squeeze of your hand. Remember, they can still hear. (See Hearing)

It is not uncommon for their eyes to stare, like they are looking through you. Sometimes they have a glazed look. If they are not blinking, liquid tears should be used to prevent the eye from drying.

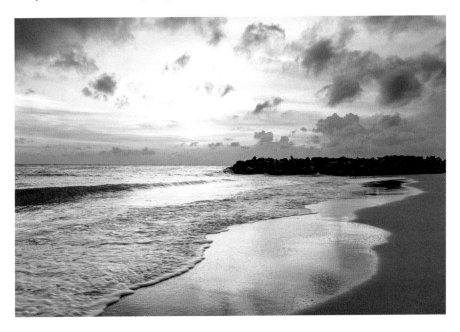

BREATHING

Respiration patterns can vary from person to person. In the latter stages of life, you may notice a breathing pattern called Cheyne-Stokes. There are several breaths and then a pause without any breaths, called apnea. The apnea may last only 5 to 10 seconds, but can be as long as a minute, especially at the very end. This pattern can come and go, so it is not always a sure sign that the end is close.

Another pattern that is common, especially once someone is comatose, is a rhythmic, labored breathing. Sometimes it can be very rapid and shallow and other times, very slow and labored. There may be a moaning with each breath. This should not be confused with pain. The moan is like singing; it helps to hold the oxygen in their lungs longer. An oscillating fan can have a calming affect on labored breathing.

Your loved one may, or may not, want to wear their oxygen. This is okay. Oxygen can be a comfort measure for some and a nuisance for others. Again, an oscillating fan may be all that is necessary.

At the end, it may appear that they are taking full in and out breaths. However, most of the breath is an out breath. The final breath is an expiration.

HEARING

A person can hear until their very last breath. Hearing can become very acute also. I have experienced deaf people hear again. I've also experienced them hearing what we were talking about in the other room! It is important to make every word be what you want them to hear. It is a great time to reminisce, look at photo albums, share stories, and especially, be kind and loving to each other. They want to know that everyone is going to be just fine when they take their last breath. When it is not possible for that "important person" to come to their bedside, call them and hold the phone to your loved ones ear so they can hear their voice. Being able to make closure with them may be just what is needed to bring them that last element of peace they need in order to let go.

Telling your loved one it is OK with you for them to go can be very hard to say, but very important. Dr. Ira Byock, in his book "Dying Well," says there are five important things to say to someone who is dying: "I love you," "I forgive you," "I know you forgive me," "Thank you," and "Goodbye." Forgiveness, not just of others, but of your self as well, is the key to all healing, including that of the spirit.

PAIN

Pain, generally, is not a symptom that death is near. If pain has been a part of your loved ones disease process, then the doctors and nurses have been evaluating it and keeping it adequately controlled. However, in the last few days, those who have been in good pain control may have their pain levels escalate and need more frequent and/or increased dosing. This last phase of the "laboring out" can be tiring and worrisome. As caregivers, we tend to take on our loved ones pain and suffering. Your Hospice nurse is always available to assist you with management of pain and other symptoms.

Again, please remember that time released tablets are **NOT** to be broken or crushed. If your loved one can no longer swallow their pills, the nurse will work with you and your doctor on an alternative means to keep their pain controlled. It is also very important **not** to stop their pain management. Should this be done, they will withdraw from their comfort and the pain can take them out of their dying process.

Occasionally, it seems there just isn't enough pain medicine to make a difference. You give more, and more, and more, and no change. This is very tiring and frustrating. My experience has me convinced that this means there is some element of spiritual or emotional component to their pain. If your loved one is still talking, ask them if something is troubling them; you might be surprised by what they tell you. Hopefully, it will be something that you can help them resolve. It may be a time for the Hospice Chaplain to make a visit.

At some point in their laboring out, most people come to terms with whatever it is that is holding them back. This may come from forgiveness of someone or of themselves, or hearing the voice of a special someone on the phone. Reminding them that it is okay to let go, to take the hand that is reaching out to them. It is honest to let them know you will be sad and miss them and that you have to let go of them too. And, reassuring them that you will be okay. Acceptance of "what is" brings peacefulness and closure. It is always nice when we can help them find their way back.

The last phase of the journey, or labor, whether it is coming into life or leaving life, can be hard work, for everyone. Some of us have short, easy labors and others, long and tiring. When the end result has come, there is a sense of relief. With birth there is usually joy; with death, a sadness. There is the saying that we should cry at birth and celebrate death. For me, these two processes, the birthing into life and the birthing out of life, remind me that everything in nature is cyclic. And, that grief and joy includes both tears and laughter. Sometimes you can be so happy that you cry. These are just two of the ways our bodies use to heal our emotions.

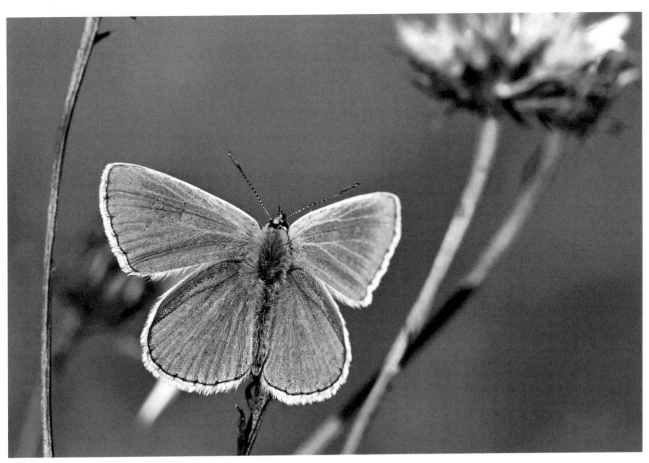

FOR CAREGIVERS

Most importantly, as caregiver, you need to take care of yourself; sleep, eat, walk, get away for short periods of time. Without you, their wish to die at home cannot be. Your Hospice volunteer is there for you and your needs.

And, above all, please remember that all of these signs and symptoms are nature's way of bringing us to the end of our life. Reassurance, guidance and support are available to you through Hospice services including bereavement follow-up. Many caregivers, widows, widowers, family members, find that joining a support group often helps them with understanding and getting through their grief. Hospices provide this service to their communities. If you are an out-of-town person experiencing grief, your nearest Hospice can help you with your bereavement issues.

The laboring out of life can be a hard job. Trusting this process as the caregiver, can be an even harder job. If you can find that trust however, you will be a lot calmer and peaceful when the end of life comes. The old saying, "Trust the process," is so true.

If you think that death is imminent or has occurred and you need someone to confirm this, call your Hospice. Always note the time that you believe the breathing stopped. Hospice can provide you with assistance. Most hospices will send a nurse out to pronounce the death or simply to be with you. They can call the doctor and mortuary, and arrange pick-up of medical equipment. They are there for you.

Again, PLEASE DO **NOT** CALL 911 for assistance unless the patient wishes were to have life sustaining measures taken. Hospice provides 24 hour on-call service.

ABOUT THE AUTHOR

Leah's work is truly her vocation. She has been assisting patients, families and caregivers since she became a nurse in 1982, graduating with a Bachelor of Science degree in Nursing from California State University Sacramento. Her work started in a cancer unit at a major hospital in Sacramento, CA, She transitioned to Home Health Care and Hospice when she realized that dying didn't need to happen in the hospital; that it could happen at home on the dying persons terms. Leah was an Oncology Certified Nurse for 12 years and then became certified as a Hospice and Palliative Care Nurse. Her years of experience have brought her many insights, one being, that people want to feel love around them when they die. It can be the love of a nurse, but mostly, it is the love of family, including pets. She says that this loving presence helps to alleviate the fear. It is impossible to experience both love and fear at the same time. It has been Leah's deepest calling to help those facing the end of life.

When Leah started with Hospice of Ukiah in 1996, she quickly found that many of her on-call phone calls were questions related to the dying process. To try and eliminate some of them, she put together a paper of the questions most commonly asked and it has been used as a handout to their Hospice families. Now she has expanded on this information and wishes to share it with others.

Leah is the proud mother of two daughters and two granddaughters. This booklet is dedicated to them: Pamela, Angela, Lily and Rebekah; plus the two other important women in her life, her late mother, Mae, and her late grandmother, Leila. And, in loving memory of her father Phil. And to all of the hundreds of patients, their families and caregivers, "they have all been my teachers." *Leah*

Disclaimer: Text written in 2011; edited in 2024.

Printed in the United States
by Baker & Taylor Publisher Services